Alive **Natural Health Guides**

Mushrooms

FOR HEALTH
AND LONGEVITY

Ken Babal, CN

books
Alive
Summertown
TENNESSEE

CONTENTS

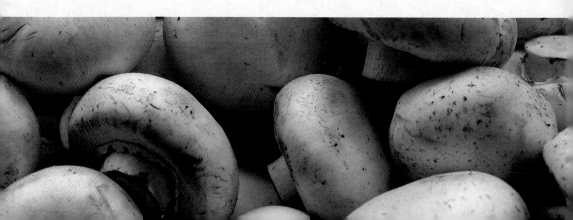

RECIPES

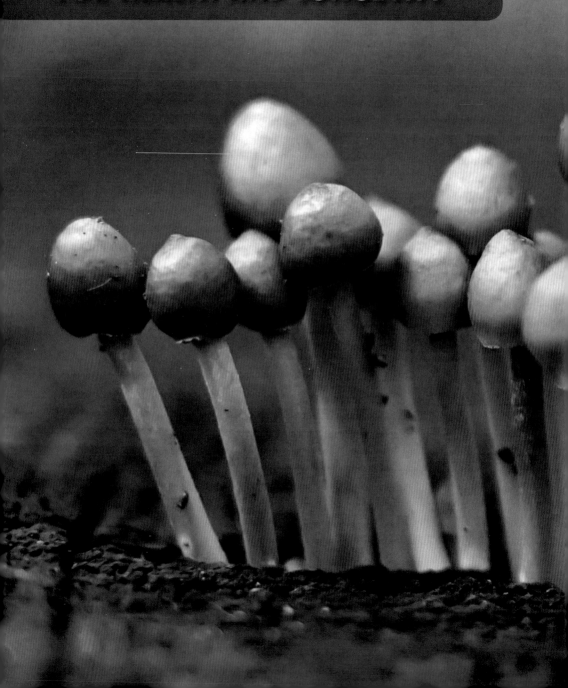

mushrooms
FOR HEALTH AND LONGEVITY

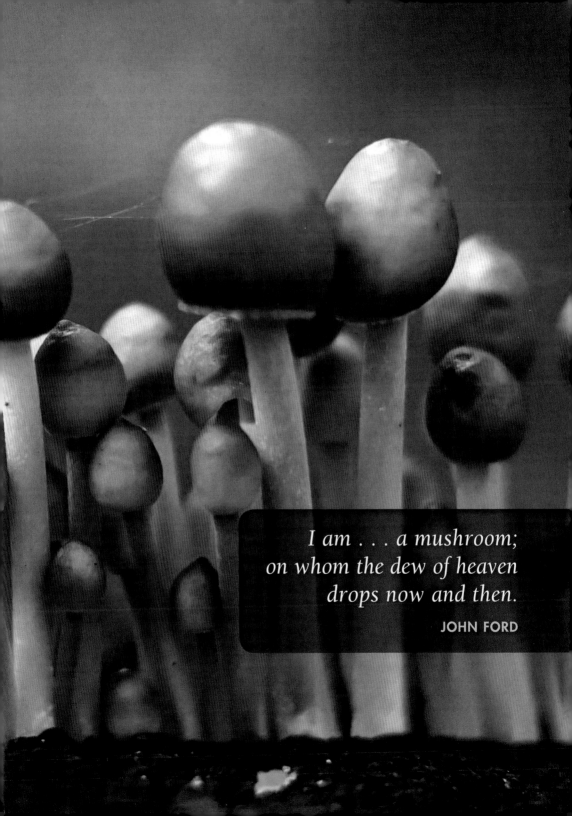

I am . . . a mushroom;
on whom the dew of heaven
drops now and then.

JOHN FORD

FUNGUS AMONG US

Mushrooms are one of the many kinds of fungi that inhabit our world. There are one hundred thousand species within the broad category of fungi, of which the penicillin mold is one, and there are thirty-eight thousand species of mushrooms. Species can differ greatly in their chemical content. For example, about fifty species of mushrooms are poisonous and another fifty demonstrate medicinal value.

The study of fungi is called mycology.

Fungi are everywhere—in the air around us, in the soil beneath our feet, in our refrigerators, and even in our bodies. The main fungus that lives in the human body is *Candida albicans.* Candida is part of the normal human flora that inhabits the intestinal tract, mouth, and skin. Like weeds in a garden, Candida can sometimes grow out of control if it is not kept in check by beneficial probiotic bacteria and yeasts.

In the United States, mushrooms are often regarded with suspicion. One reason is that some varieties are poisonous. Another reason is that in the 1960s, "magic mushrooms" were used to produce hallucinogenic trips similar to those produced by LSD. In addition, because mushrooms appear to have properties that are similar to those of cancer—they are like parasites and fast growing—even early cancer researchers were skeptical of their potential medicinal benefits.

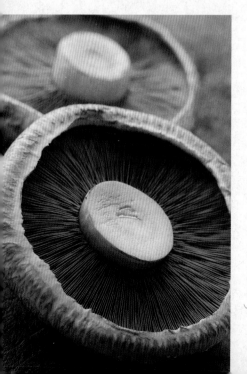

Some people might feel uneasy when they think of mushrooms as fungi. After all, the word "fungus" can bring to mind unappealing thoughts of athlete's foot, mildew in dirty shower stalls, moldy fruit, and white fuzz on stale bread. But the more you learn about mushrooms, the more you will appreciate their ecological, gastronomic, and medicinal value. You might even become a passionate mycologist and grow your own.

The Third Kingdom

Mushrooms and other fungi have been called "the third kingdom." Being neither plant nor animal, they are a world unto themselves.

ANCIENT GIANTS

Mushrooms are among the oldest and largest organisms on the planet. A honey mushroom (*Armillaria ostoyae*) was discovered under 2,200 acres (about 3.5 square miles) of the Malheur National Forest in eastern Oregon. It eclipsed the previous record of a mushroom discovered in 1992, which covered 1,500 acres in Washington State.

Fungi have been on earth for billions of years. In Saudi Arabia, scientists have identified a twenty-foot-tall fossil as an enormous mushroom. Now extinct for 350 million years, it was probably the largest organism in the world at one time.

Mushrooms resemble plants in that they have cell walls and cannot move on their own. Yet mushrooms are not really plants as we generally think of them. Instead of containing cellulose in their cell walls, they contain chitin, a substance also found in the exoskeleton of shellfish. Their genetic makeup is more similar to that of humans and animals than to plants. (We share about 30 percent of our DNA with mushrooms.)

Mushrooms are living, breathing organisms. While plants absorb carbon dioxide and liberate oxygen, mushrooms mimic human respiration by capturing oxygen and exhaling carbon dioxide. But unlike humans who need light and fresh food, mushrooms feed on moist organic matter in deep shade.

Mushrooms also differ from plants in that they contain no chlorophyll and cannot manufacture food energy from the sun. They emerge at night and obtain their energy from decaying plant matter. Instead of calories from solar energy, they are said to provide lunar energy, which some experts believe stimulates imagination and intuition.

Fungi, either single celled or multicellular, feed by directly absorbing nutrients. The fungi first secrete enzymes that dissolve organic substances, then they absorb this food through thin cell walls. In our forests, mushrooms perform the essential ecological function of recycling leaves and dead plants. About 85 percent of all plants, particularly trees, have developed a symbiotic relationship with mushrooms. Leaves and other organisms that are decomposed by mushrooms nourish the trees and create space for plants and animals by breaking down dead trees.

CULINARY VALUE OF MUSHROOMS

Mushrooms have been valued throughout the world as both food and medicine. About seven hundred species, many of which have been cultivated since the nineteenth century, are used for food. In the United States, however, mushrooms are often underrated. The button mushroom (*Agaricus bisporus*) is the most common variety sold here. Only recently have some of the more exotic varieties appeared in U.S. markets. Mushrooms such as enoki, oyster, porcini, portobello, and shiitake are now popular in gourmet cuisine and available year-round.

For centuries, Asians and Europeans have appreciated the culinary value of wild mushrooms, which can be hard to come by. They are gathered and sold by experts who build their businesses on the safety of their product, since some species are poisonous and can make a person deathly ill. Searching for wild mushrooms can be as fun as an Easter egg hunt and very profitable too. Hard-to-find varieties can fetch up to $650 a pound. Some of these mycological trophies include chanterelle, fried chicken mushroom, king bolete (porcini), morel, and truffle.

Mushrooms are cultivated commercially in limestone caves, dark cellars, or specially constructed houses in which humidity and temperature are carefully maintained. In the United States, 65 percent of all cultivated mushrooms are grown in Kennett Square, Pennsylvania. Known as the "mushroom capital of the world," Kennett Square has the highest concentration of mushroom farms, including Creekside Mushrooms and Phillips Mushroom Farms. Phillips is the largest producer of specialty mushrooms, including cremini, Lion's Mane, portobello (one of the biggest sellers), and trumpet.

WILD, RARE, AND COSTLY

The truffle is the most prized fungi of all. It is a rare delicacy that is reserved for the rich or used only on very special occasions. An Italian white truffle that weighed 3.3 pounds sold for over $300,000 at auction. Because of their high cost, truffles are often sliced thinly and served as part of other dishes.

After truffles, morels are perhaps the rarest and costliest of the wild fungi. They have distinctive wrinkled, conical caps and a wonderfully earthy, smoky flavor. They cannot be cultivated, so fresh morels are extremely hard to come by. They are most likely to be found dried.

NUTRITIONAL VALUE OF MUSHROOMS

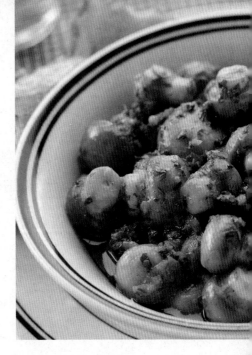

Many people mistakenly believe that mushrooms contribute little to health. Although a mushroom's specific nutritional content is determined by how it is cultivated, mushrooms are generally rich sources of essential amino acids, minerals, and vitamins, including thiamin (B_1), riboflavin (B_2), and niacin (B_3). In addition, mushrooms are high in fiber and low in calories, making them the perfect food for people who want to lose weight.

Mushrooms are unique in that they are the only vegan source of vitamin D (other than sunlight and ultraviolet light exposure). They contain abundant quantities of the provitamin ergosterol, which is not found in vegetables. Ergosterol is converted to active vitamin D in the body, just as beta-carotene in fruits and vegetables is converted to vitamin A. Mushrooms also contain small amounts of preformed vitamin D_2 (ergocalciferol). A three-ounce serving of brown button mushrooms provides about 16 IU (international units), which is 4 percent of the Daily Value. (The vitamin D content of a food is not required to be listed on food packaging unless the food has been fortified with this nutrient.)

Research shows that ergosterol in button mushrooms can be rapidly converted to active vitamin D_2 when mushrooms are exposed to ultraviolet (UV) light before or after harvesting. This process greatly increases their vitamin D content. Mushrooms react to sunlight in the same way as

THE NEW MEAT

Because certain mushrooms and fungi are high in protein, they can be processed into meat substitutes. A fungal-based product line called Quorn is one of the most popular meatless brands in Europe. Quorn products are made from a mycoprotein that comes from a mold called *Fusarium venenatum*, whose fibrous fungal structure imparts a meatlike texture. People in the United Kingdom alone consume over five hundred thousand Quorn-based meals every day.

humans and produce a totally natural form of vitamin D.

Mushrooms that have been exposed to UV light are now being sold commercially in the United States. Monterey Mushrooms offers UV-exposed white and brown button mushrooms as well as portobello mushrooms. Dole received a Good Housekeeping Award for their vitamin D portobello mushrooms. A three-ounce serving of UV-exposed mushrooms provides 100 percent of the daily value for vitamin D.

Many of us are familiar with vitamin D's role in keeping our bones strong. However, new and exciting research suggests that vitamin D reduces tumor growth, lowers cancer risk, and reduces the risk of diabetes and multiple sclerosis. New findings show that many American adults do not spend enough time outside to receive the UV exposure they need to produce ample vitamin D. The problem is especially acute in winter. This is a good reason to eat more mushrooms.

In addition to essential nutrients and vitamins, mushrooms contain many compounds that have protective and therapeutic value against certain diseases. One of these is beta-glucan, a complex carbohydrate, or polysaccharide, composed of glucose sugar molecules that are strung together. Scientific studies show that glucans are largely responsible for medicinal mushrooms' antitumor properties and immunologic activity.

Although we generally think of carbohydrates as providing energy to bodily cells, research reveals that some are involved in molecular recognition. Specifically, cell-surface carbohydrates help to facilitate communication between cells in certain kinds of interactions. Receptors for beta-glucans can be found on macrophages, the large white blood cells that engage in phagocytosis (the engulfing and ingestion of bacteria, foreign particles, and tissue debris by phagocytes). When macrophages are activated by beta-glucan, they in turn trigger a cascade of events that stimulate the immune system.

Beta-glucans are also found in other foods, including oats and yeast. However, their chemical structures and effects are often different from those of the beta-glucans in medicinal mushrooms.

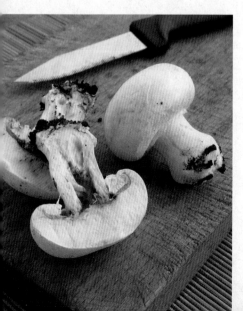

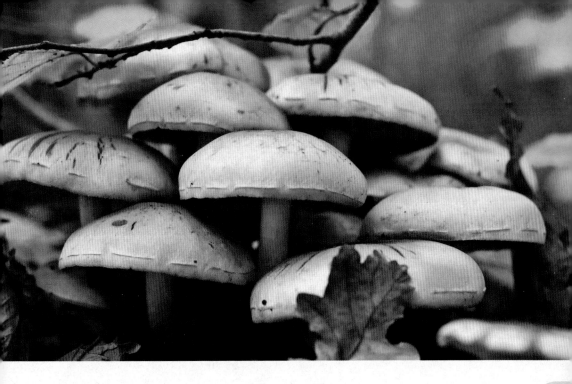

MEDICINAL VALUE OF MUSHROOMS

For thousands of years people have consumed mushrooms such as maitake, reishi, shiitake, and others to maintain and improve health, preserve youth, and increase longevity. In ancient China and Japan these mushrooms were highly valued and reserved only for emperors or royal families.

Reishi is among the top-ranked ingredients in traditional Chinese medicine (TCM). Shiitake is also highly regarded and is said to boost *chi*, or life energy. In Japanese herbal medicine (*kampo*), maitake is used as a treatment for a variety of conditions and as a tonic to strengthen the body and improve overall health.

Today, mushrooms are still considered the greatest of tonics, promoting overall well-being and vibrant health. In natural food and supplement stores, mushrooms are carving out their own niche as dietary supplements apart from herbs and vitamins.

HAVE MUSHROOMS, WILL TRAVEL

Ötzi the Iceman, who lived 5,300 years ago and whose frozen remains were found in 1991 on the border of Austria and Italy, carried three kinds of mushrooms. This remarkable find suggests that he considered mushrooms essential during his trek over the Alps.

Scientific studies show that certain mushrooms enhance the immune system and have potent antitumor properties that make them promising cancer treatments. You might be surprised to learn that protein-bound polysaccharide (PSK), a best-selling anticancer drug in Europe and Japan, is a mushroom extract. In numerous experiments and clinical trials, mushrooms have also demonstrated antiallergenic, antibacterial, anti-inflammatory, and antiviral actions, and an ability to sensitize cells to insulin.

In TCM, mushrooms are recommended to neutralize the toxic effects of excess meat eating. Studies have shown that certain mushrooms support liver function, which may improve the body's detoxification processes. Many natural-health practitioners know that if the health of the liver can be improved, overall health will benefit, since the liver is the largest organ within the body and performs hundreds of vital functions.

TCM recognizes that health depends upon the body's capacity to maintain equilibrium (*yin-yang* balance) by adapting to changing conditions. Medicinal mushrooms are beneficial to this process because they are adaptogenic, which means they help us adapt to various types of stress by normalizing altered bodily conditions. For example, adaptogens help us maintain a normal body weight and healthful levels of blood pressure, blood sugar, and cholesterol. Medicinal mushrooms also are tonifying (a tonic is a substance that strengthens or invigorates glands and organs or the entire organism).

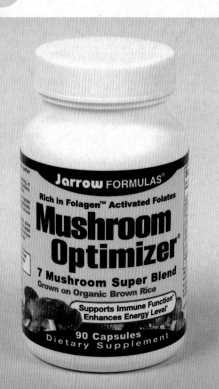

MUSHROOMS AS MEDICINE

Mushrooms are natural medicines that help protect us from the health challenges of the twenty-first century. It makes good sense to include them as a regular part of the diet. People who want more powerful, consistent effects or do not enjoy eating mushrooms should consider mushroom supplements. In some cases, mushrooms are not edible and can only be taken as supplements. Reishi, for example, is too tough and woody to eat. There are a number of active ingredients in mushrooms that are obtained by alcohol extraction or methods other than simple hot water extraction. The best way to obtain these ingredients is to take standardized liquid or dried mushroom extracts.

Table 1 shows the descriptions and medicinal properties of the best-known healing mushrooms. If you are unable to decide which one might be best for you, look for a mushroom combination formula, or try alternating your use of different mushroom supplements.

Agaricus *Mushroom of God*

Agaricus blazei grows on the grasslands of Florida and South Carolina. However, its main habitat is the mountainous regions of southeastern Brazil, where it is called *Cogmelo de Dues* (Mushroom of God). Interest in this mushroom's medicinal effects grew when it was discovered that many adults in this region experienced a much lower incidence of disease and lived longer than average.

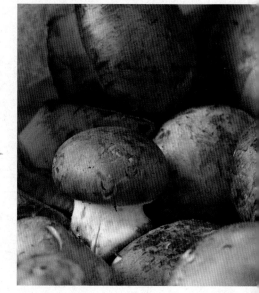

The cultivation of Agaricus was pioneered by Japanese mycologists who took specimens from Brazil back to Japan, where it now enjoys superstar status. Its medicinal actions include counteracting or preventing tumors, fighting viruses, lowering cholesterol, regulating blood sugar levels, and enhancing immunity. Its reputation as a longevity aid is supported by studies of laboratory mice that show Agaricus prolongs their life span, revitalizes tissue, and positively affects metabolism and digestion. Human studies have not yet been completed.

Agaricus contains compounds that inhibit aromatase, an enzyme responsible for a key step in the biosynthesis of estrogens. Because estrogens promote certain cancers and other diseases, aromatase inhibitors are frequently used to

TABLE 1: Therapeutic applications of medicinal mushrooms

THERAPEUTIC APPLICATIONS	TYPES OF MEDICINAL MUSHROOMS										
	Agaricus	Chaga	Cordyceps	Coriolus	Enoki	Lion's Mane	Maitake	Meshima	Reishi	Shiitake	Tremella
Antioxidant	✔	✔	✔	✔	✔		✔		✔		
Antiallergy	✔								✔	✔	
Athletics			✔			✔					
Cancer or antitumor	✔	✔	✔	✔	✔	✔	✔	✔	✔	✔	✔
Cardiovascular			✔						✔		
Dementia						✔			✔		
Diabetes	✔		✔				✔		✔	✔	
Digestive			✔			✔					
Hepatitis	✔		✔	✔			✔		✔	✔	✔
High blood pressure			✔		✔		✔		✔	✔	✔
High cholesterol	✔		✔		✔		✔		✔	✔	✔
Immune enhancement	✔	✔	✔	✔	✔	✔	✔	✔	✔	✔	✔
Infection	✔	✔	✔	✔			✔		✔	✔	
Inflammation		✔	✔	✔					✔		✔
Kidney disease			✔								
Nervous system			✔			✔			✔		
Radiation or chemo adjunct			✔				✔		✔	✔	✔
Respiratory			✔			✔			✔		
Sexual function			✔								
Weight loss							✔				✔

treat those diseases. The compounds in Agaricus that inhibit aromatase have great potential for breast cancer prevention and treatment.

Chaga *Siberian Superstar*

Chaga (*Inonotus obliquus*) has received wide acclaim as a medicinal mushroom ever since the Nobel Prize-winning Russian novelist Aleksandr Solzhenitsyn introduced it in his 1968 novel, *Cancer Ward*. He described chaga as a "birch tree mushroom" with remarkable health benefits and spoke of a cancerous lesion that was cured by its application.

In Russian medicine, a tea made from chaga is used as a diuretic, to treat ulcers and tuberculosis, and to counteract or prevent tumors. Chaga gained attention when it was observed that very few cancer cases were reported in the health records of residents of a rural district of Russia near Moscow. This low cancer rate is attributed to the custom of drinking a hot-water decoction of chaga, because it is less expensive than black tea. This regional custom has continued for centuries.

In scientific studies, chaga has demonstrated a variety of beneficial cardiovascular effects and a range of actions that support the immune system, including the activation of B cells and macrophages. In a comparison study of mushrooms' effects on free radicals (unstable molecules that cause aging and disease), chaga exhibited the strongest fighting response.

In the 1950s, chaga was approved in Russia as an anticancer drug and is reportedly successful in treating breast, cervical, lung, and stomach cancers.

Unlike other mushrooms, chaga does not produce a fruiting body with a characteristic stem and cap. Rather, it is an irregular, lumpy growth that develops under tree bark and eventually pushes the bark away from the tree. Chaga's medicinal properties are concentrated in the sclerotium, which is a hardened mass of the mycelia, or rootlike structures that grow beneath the surface. A Japanese study of laboratory mice confirmed that chaga sclerotia possessed antitumor and hypoglycemic effects.

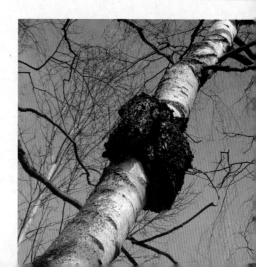

Chaga also contains the triterpene betulin, a subject of much confusion and misinformation. White birch trees, on which chaga grows, are reported to contain betulin as well as betulinic acid. Studies show that betulinic acid has anti-HIV, anti-inflammatory, antimalarial, and antitumor activities. However, betulin does not normally convert to betulinic acid, and there are no reports of betulin having the same biologic activities as betulinic acid. Furthermore, neither betulin nor betulinic acid dissolves in water, so it is doubtful that either is responsible for the health benefits of chaga tea.

With these facts in mind, Cun Zhuang, PhD, one of the original chaga researchers, developed a proprietary extract that is made from Siberian chaga sclerotia. The extract is believed to offer powerful antioxidants and benefit the cardiovascular and immune systems. The dried extract comes in tablets and is sourced from wildcrafted chaga mushrooms, which grow naturally on birch trees in Siberia.

Cordyceps *Caterpillar Fungus*

Cordyceps sinensis is a rare, potent, and highly treasured mushroom that was once used exclusively in the Chinese emperor's palace. It grows as a parasite on the larvae of a moth, mummifies the caterpillar, and sprouts the mushroom fruit off the caterpillar's head, before poking through the soil. More than 1,500 years ago, Chinese herders noticed that their animals became more energetic after eating these caterpillar mushrooms.

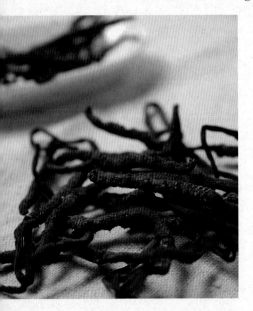

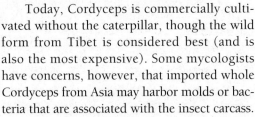

Today, Cordyceps is commercially cultivated without the caterpillar, though the wild form from Tibet is considered best (and is also the most expensive). Some mycologists have concerns, however, that imported whole Cordyceps from Asia may harbor molds or bacteria that are associated with the insect carcass.

Cordyceps strengthens lung power and is highly regarded in China as a tonic for those recovering from illness, an operation, or giving birth. In these instances, it helps patients recover physical energy while improving appetite and protecting the body from infection. Throughout Asia, Cordyceps is used to treat fungal and yeast infections.

A group of Japanese researchers presented a paper showing that an aqueous Cordyceps extract dilated the aorta, the largest artery in

Cordyceps is a good choice for those who require energy for physical work. It is used by world-class athletes and has made international sports headlines. At the Chinese National Games in 1993, a team of nine Chinese women runners shattered nine world records, breaking the record for the 10,000-meter run by an unprecedented forty-two seconds. The athletes attributed their success to an intense training regimen and the use of Cordyceps.

the body, by 40 percent under stress. Dilation increases blood flow, which can benefit muscles that are pushed to their maximum, thus greatly enhancing endurance.

Research has also focused on how Cordyceps lowers cholesterol and enhances immune function. The mushroom has general cardiotonic properties, which means it tends to increase the heart's muscle tone, and inhibits cholesterol from being deposited in the aorta.

Cordyceps contains various compounds that have antitumor and immunologic activities. In test tube experiments, Cordyceps inhibits the proliferation of human leukemia cells. Some researchers have suggested that it can be used in the treatment of adult leukemia. The U.S. National Institutes of Health is currently screening a Cordyceps compound as a possible treatment for leukemia.

17

Cordyceps is considered one of the best sexual tonics, although it is not quick acting. It is commonly recommended for frigidity, impotence, infertility, and sexual malaise. A clinical study of sexually dysfunctional men found that 64 percent improved in performance after ingesting 1 gram of Cordyceps per day.

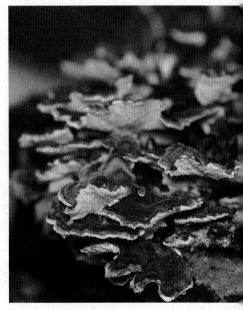

Coriolus *Turkey Tail*

Coriolus versicolor (also known as *Trametes versicolor*) may be the most studied medicinal mushroom of all. The immunologic activities of Coriolus and its constituents have been extensively studied in Japan since the mid-1970s, and it has been the subject of over four hundred clinical studies. Its common name, "turkey tail," is derived from its multicolored, fan-shaped fruiting bodies that grow in overlapping clusters.

In traditional Chinese medicine, Coriolus is used to clear dampness and phlegm, heal lung disorders, increase energy, strengthen the physique, and treat chronic conditions. It is used to treat liver ailments, including hepatitis B and chronic active hepatitis, and infection and inflammation of the digestive, upper respiratory, and urinary tracts. It is also used for strengthening the immune response.

Coriolus is the source of one of the all-time best-selling cancer drugs. Protein-bound polysaccharide, known as PSK, which also goes by the brand name Krestin, is sold mainly in Europe and Japan. Two other substances extracted from the mushroom, PSP and VSP, are being studied as possible complementary cancer treatments. Clinical trials suggest that PSK can be used to treat a wide variety of cancers by increasing survival rates and lengthening intervals between disease, without causing major side effects. PSK is used as an adjunct to radiation and chemotherapy and is most commonly administered by injection.

PSK has potent antimicrobial activity against *Candida albicans*, *Escherichia coli*, and *Listeria*. The mushroom uses these substances to protect itself against rot. Its traditional use in soups and teas was well warranted for this benefit. One other important feature of Coriolus is the ability of its protein-bound polysaccharides to stimulate superoxide dismutase (SOD). SOD is the body's most powerful antioxidant enzyme that neutralizes free radicals. (Free radicals are unstable molecules that are destructive to cells and cause deterioration.)

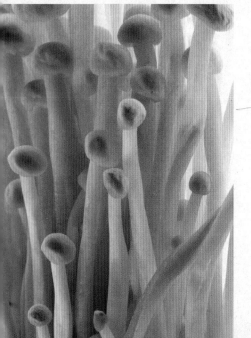

Enoki *Golden Needle*

Enoki (*Flammulina velutipes*) mushrooms are long, thin, white mushrooms that are often used in Asian cuisine. They have a crisp texture and are a good choice for grilling or adding to salads or soups. Before grilling, simply leave the enoki mushrooms in a bunch and baste them with mirin, oil, and soy sauce.

Research on enoki is limited compared to that on other medicinal mushrooms. However, studies show that enoki strongly stimulates cellular immunity and has potent antitumor properties. In addition, the mushroom contains compounds that lower cholesterol and blood pressure levels. Enoki contains polysaccharides that significantly increase cellular nitric oxide, an important messenger molecule in the body that is needed to control high blood pressure.

The stalk of enoki mushrooms contains a protein known as FVE, which interacts with immune system cells, resulting in the production of a number of immune system messengers (cytokines). In one research study, oral administration of FVE to mice with liver tumors reduced the size of their tumors and significantly increased their life spans. Further enoki research is aimed at the possible development of pharmaceutical products for cancer prevention and treatment. Scientists suggest that enoki might be effective against lymphoma, melanoma, and cancers of the breast and prostate.

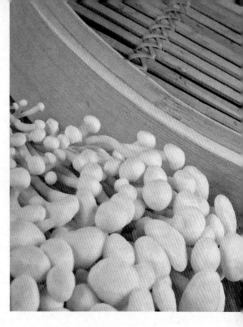

A researcher with the National Cancer Institute of Tokyo conducted an epidemiological study of enoki growers in Japan and found that their families had substantially lower cancer rates than were found in the surrounding communities or the country overall.

Enoki contains potent antioxidants that scavenge free radicals and are more effective than either sodium ascorbate (vitamin C) or alpha-tocopherol (vitamin E) as a preservative. It's important to note that antioxidants perform similarly in the human body. By slowing the oxidation of fats, antioxidants are able to inhibit deterioration and aging of tissues and organs.

Lion's Mane *Mushroom for the Brain*

Lion's Mane (*Hericium erinaceus*) is an edible mushroom that is widely distributed in Japan and China. Its name comes from its beautiful white spines, which resemble a lion's mane or icicles.

Scientific studies performed in Asia confirm Lion's Mane traditional use as a tonic for the cardiovascular, nervous, and respiratory systems. One variety of the mushroom is marketed as a remedy for gastric and duodenal ulcers and chronic gastritis. In traditional Chinese medicine, Lion's Mane is used to promote good digestion, strength, and vigor and to prevent gastrointestinal cancer. Its beta-glucan composition is very similar to that of some of the most potent anticancer mushrooms. In addition, a hot-water

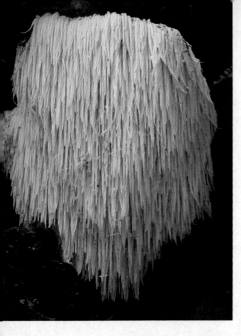

extract made from Lion's Mane is considered a health tonic and sports beverage. Most important, Japanese studies show that Lion's Mane is able to regenerate neurons by stimulating production of nerve growth factor (NGF).

NGF belongs to a family of proteins that play a part in the maintenance, survival, and regeneration of neurons in adults. As we age, NGF declines, resulting in less efficient brain functioning. In mice, its absence leads to a condition resembling Alzheimer's disease. In 1986, two scientists won the Nobel Prize in Physiology or Medicine for the discovery and isolation of NGF. Since its discovery, researchers have been exploring its medical potential. But because NGF is unable to cross the blood-brain barrier, it cannot be administered as an oral drug. Accordingly, scientists directed their attention to finding bioactive compounds with a low molecular weight that could penetrate the blood-brain barrier and be taken orally to induce synthesis of NGF within the brain.

A breakthrough occurred when a Japanese research team discovered a class of compounds called hericenones in Lion's Mane that stimulate production of NGF, causing neurons to regrow. These compounds offer great potential for repairing neurological damage, improving intelligence and reflexes, and even preventing and treating Alzheimer's disease. What's more, hericenones are the first active substances found in plants to induce NGF synthesis. Other known compounds in Lion's Mane, as well as some yet to be identified, are also believed to be bioactive.

Amyloban, a fat-soluble substance isolated from Lion's Mane, was found to protect against neuronal cell death caused by toxic beta-amyloid peptide. Beta-amyloid peptide is the main component of plaque that develops in the brains of patients with Alzheimer's disease, causing destruction of neurons as the disease progresses.

A study at Chinese Pharmaceutical University compared a Lion's Mane extract (Amycenone) standardized to contain hericenones (0.5%) and amyloban (6%) with donepezil (Aricept), a common Alzheimer's drug. One hundred rats were injected with beta-amyloid peptide to create a dementia similar to Alzheimer's. The rats were then divided into groups to receive either Lion's Mane extract or the drug once a day for four weeks. At the fourth week, learning and memory-related behavior were assessed for seven consecutive days. Results showed that the rats treated with the mushroom extract performed a water maze test as well as or better than the mice treated with the Alzheimer's drug, depending on the dosage of the extract. After completing the behavioral test, all rats were sacrificed for pathological examination to determine the NGF content in the brain. It was found that the rats who received Lion's Mane extract produced significantly more NGF.

A clinical study using Lion's Mane was conducted to investigate its effectiveness against dementia in a rehabilitative hospital in Japan. The study consisted of fifty patients (average age seventy-five) in the experimental group and fifty controls (average age seventy-seven). Seven of the patients in the experimental group suffered from different types of dementia. The patients in this group received 5 grams of dried mushroom per day in their soup for six months. All patients were evaluated before and after the treatment period for their functional independence measure (FIM), which is an international evaluation standard of independence in physical capabilities (bathing or showering, dressing, eating, evacuating, walking, and so on) and of perceptive capabilities (communication, expression, memory, problem solving, and understanding). Results showed that after six months of taking Lion's Mane, six out of seven patients experienced improvements in their overall FIM score. Notably, three bedridden patients were able to get up to eat meals after being treated with Lion's Mane.

Another study, this time a double-blind, placebo-controlled study, demonstrated that Lion's Mane is effective in patients diagnosed with mild cognitive impairment. A group of thirty Japanese men and women ages fifty to eighty was split randomly into two. One group was given Lion's Mane and the other a placebo. The subjects in the Lion's Mane group took four 250-milligram tablets, three times per day, for sixteen weeks. At weeks eight, twelve, and sixteen of the trial, the Lion's Mane group showed significantly increased scores on a cognitive-function scale compared with the placebo group. It was observed that the group's scores increased with the duration of intake. However, four weeks after the patients stopped taking the supplement, the scores decreased significantly. Laboratory tests showed no adverse effects of Lion's Mane. These studies are very encouraging, and more extensive clinical studies are currently under way at other hospitals.

Presently, there is no cure for Alzheimer's disease, and conventional treatments only address the symptoms of the disease. About one in ten people over age sixty-five are diagnosed with the condition. More troubling, half of those who make it into their eighties are expected to contract Alzheimer's. It has been suggested that NGF may be used to treat Alzheimer's disease. For this reason, compounds in Lion's Mane are attracting great attention for preventing and treating various types of dementia. An effective way to reduce the risk of Alzheimer's and other types of dementia might be the daily intake of foods or dietary supplements that stimulate NGF and inhibit the toxicity of beta-amyloid peptide. It is now known that beta-amyloid begins to accumulate in the brain ten to fifteen years before the onset of dementia.

Maitake *King of Mushrooms*

The scientific name for maitake, *Grifola frondosa*, is derived from the common name of a mushroom in Italy and refers to a mythical half-lion, half-eagle beast. Maitake is indigenous to the northeastern part of Japan. The mushroom has a rippling appearance, has no caps, and grows in clusters at the foot of oak trees. To the Japanese, this conveys an image of dancing butterflies, thus the name *maitake*, which means "dancing mushroom." Others say that maitake is so named because people who found it deep in the mountains would dance with joy because of its delicious taste and wonderful health benefits.

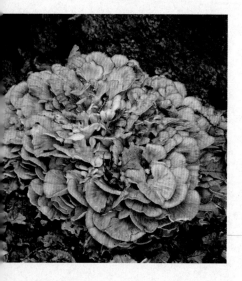

Maitake has some unique characteristics. It is the only edible mushroom in the Monkey's Bench family, which is known to enhance immunity. Maitake is a giant, often reaching twenty inches at the base. A single cluster can weigh as much as one hundred pounds. Because of its large size and amazing health benefits, it has earned an additional nickname: "the king of mushrooms."

Maitake excels in treating conditions of excess, whether it is excess blood pressure, body weight, cholesterol, or triglycerides. It may also be the best choice for enhancing immunity and inhibiting tumor growth. Most immunity and cancer research favors maitake D-fraction, the protein-bound beta-glucan extract discovered in

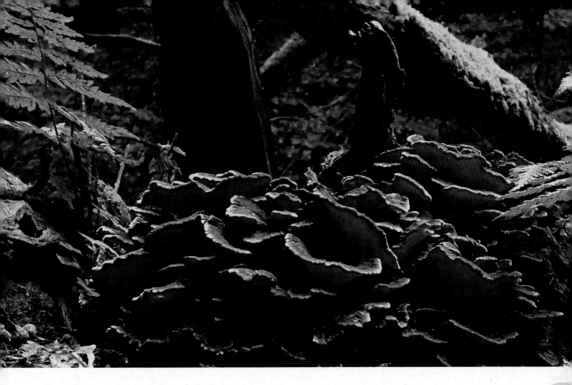

Japan and standardized by Cun Zhuang, PhD. Maitake D-fraction activates the body's immune cells, including T cells, B cells, macrophages, natural killer (NK) cells, and other vital components of cellular immunity. One study compared D-fraction with mitomycin-C (MMC), one of the strongest and most widely used chemotherapeutic drugs, which has very severe side effects. With just a small dose, the maitake extract produced an 80 percent shrinkage in tumors in mice compared to a 45 percent shrinkage produced by the MMC. When the two agents were combined in half-doses, an astonishing 98 percent shrinkage was achieved in fourteen days, demonstrating an apparent synergy.

During the feudal era of Japan, maitake had monetary value and was exchanged for the same weight in silver by local lords who in turn offered it to the shogun, *the national leader.*

In Japan, a clinical trial was performed to investigate the effect of D-fraction against various advanced cancers. The 165 patients who participated in the study were between the ages of twenty-five and sixty-five and were diagnosed with stage III or stage IV cancer. Patients were given

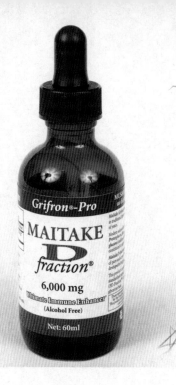

maitake D-fraction in addition to tablets made from whole maitake mushroom powder, while others received chemotherapy along with the maitake supplements.

Tumor regression or significant symptom improvements were observed among eleven of fifteen breast cancer patients, twelve of eighteen lung cancer patients, and seven of fifteen liver cancer patients. When the maitake therapies were taken with chemotherapy, these response rates improved by 12 to 18 percent. A number of patients were diagnosed as stage I after previously being diagnosed as stage III. In addition, some drastic remissions were seen. An egg-sized brain tumor in a forty-four-year-old man completely disappeared after he took the maitake D-fraction for four months. Most patients taking maitake claimed improvement of overall symptoms even when tumor regression was not observed. Although this was not a blind, placebo-controlled study, results suggest that breast, liver, and lung cancers are more favorably affected by maitake treatment than cancers of the blood (leukemia), bone, or stomach.

This study also demonstrates that maitake has a synergistic effect with chemotherapy for all types of cancer. In some cases, maitake treatment alone was almost as effective as combination therapy. In addition, many severe side effects of chemotherapy were ameliorated when maitake was included with conventional treatment. Hair loss, leukopenia (deficiency of white blood cells), and nausea were alleviated in 90 percent of patients. Pain reduction was also reported by 83 percent of patients. Authors of this study concluded that maitake improves the immune system and helps to maintain quality of life for patients, resulting in possible remission of cancer without side effects.

At the forefront of cancer research is the study of apoptosis. Apoptosis is cell death programmed by a specific set of so-called suicide genes. Scientists have discovered that all cells, including cancer cells, have the potential to self-destruct. Researchers at New York Medical College found that maitake D-fraction has strong apoptosis-inducing activity against prostate cancer cells *in vitro*.

Maitake D-fraction can also be taken by healthy individuals for protection against less serious immune deficiencies, such as colds and flu. Drops or tablets are especially helpful during cold and flu season. It has been demonstrated in cell cultures that macrophages stimulated with maitake extract inhibit the growth of influenza A virus. In many cases, macrophages are the first line of defense, responding rapidly and creating the environment for a total immune response. The anti-influenza benefit is the result of increased production of tumor necrosis factor-alpha, which is an immune system mes-

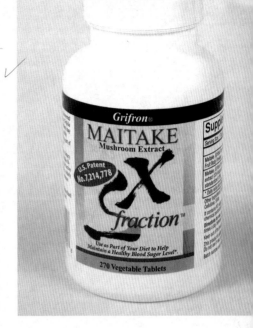

senger that has the ability to kill tumor cells and also plays a role in the body's inflammatory response and resistance to pathogens.

The success of D-fraction, both clinically and experimentally, has inspired more research to identify other bioactive compounds in maitake. American and Japanese research culminated in the identification and isolation of a glycoprotein called SX-fraction. Studies demonstrate that the compound supports glucose metabolism by enhancing insulin sensitivity, or the body's response to glucose. Research has shown that SX-fraction is a completely different compound than D-fraction because it can enhance insulin sensitivity and improve blood sugar control.

In experiments conducted at Georgetown University, SX-fraction reduced levels of fasting blood glucose, blood pressure, and body weight in genetically obese and diabetic rats. The extract also prevented hypertensive rats on a high-sugar diet from developing insulin resistance, or reduced sensitivity to insulin. Furthermore, a clinical study found that type 2 diabetics who took SX-fraction for two months were able to significantly reduce their fasting blood glucose, body weight, insulin, and triglycerides.

Maitake SX-fraction was evaluated in women with polycystic ovaries, a condition in which the ovaries do not produce eggs. The extract was chosen because insulin resistance is believed to be the underlying cause of the disorder. In the study, patients were randomly assigned to take either SX-fraction or a traditional Chinese herbal formula frequently prescribed by Japanese gynecologists. After six months, ovulation was observed in seventeen

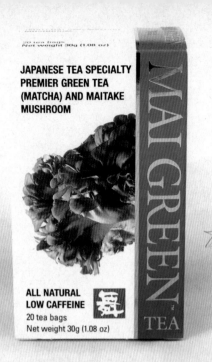

of thirty-six menstrual cycles in the SX-fraction group compared to eight out of thirty-six in the group receiving the herbal treatment. The superiority of SX-fraction was evident as early as three months into the trial. Results strongly suggest that maitake SX-fraction may help normalize menstruation, ovulation, and insulin resistance in women with polycystic ovaries.

Since insulin resistance is a prominent feature of polycystic ovary syndrome (PCOS), insulin-sensitizing drugs are often used to induce ovulation. One clinical study compared the effects of SX-fraction with clomiphene citrate, a common drug used to treat PCOS. In this study, patients were assigned to receive either the drug, SX-fraction, or a combination of both.

At the end of the trial, ovulation rates were 77 percent in subjects treated with SX-fraction and 94 percent in those receiving the drug. A significant finding was that six out of eight women who failed to respond to clomiphene alone ovulated when the drug was combined with SX-fraction. The study suggests that maitake SX-fraction alone may induce ovulation in PCOS patients and may also be useful as an adjunct for patients who fail to respond to drug treatment.

Maintaining a healthy blood sugar level is an important consideration for controlling weight. With steep fluctuations in the blood sugar level, we are more inclined to store body fat. The insulin-sensitizing glycoprotein in maitake, along with its high fiber content, makes it a useful supplement for managing weight. Fiber helps to prevent constipation by holding moisture in the bowel and increasing peristalsis, the involuntary contractions that push matter through the intestines. Results of animal research show that the water content of the stool is significantly increased after feeding with maitake powder.

Maitake's antiobesity activity has been studied in both animals and humans. The results of tests with overweight rats indicate that after eighteen weeks, those fed unheated maitake powder lost weight, whereas controls gained weight. In a human study conducted at a Tokyo clinic, patients who were given maitake supplements lost weight. Thirty patients were given twenty 500-milligram tablets of maitake powder daily for a period of two months with no change in their regular diets. All the patients lost between seven and twenty-six pounds, with an

A study published in the *International Journal of Cancer* reported that women who include plenty of mushrooms in their diets have a 64 percent lower risk of developing breast cancer. The study of over two thousand Chinese women found that the more mushrooms they consumed, the lower their risk of breast cancer. The mushroom eaters who also consumed green tea regularly reduced their risk by nearly 90 percent.

average loss of eleven to thirteen pounds. One doctor speculated that patients would have continued to lose weight if they had continued the program beyond the two months.

Meshima *Woman's Island*

Meshima (*Phellinus linteus*), literally meaning "woman's island," is a mushroom that grows on mulberry trees on an island with the same name located southwest of Japan. Meshima has been used as a traditional medicine in China, Japan, Korea, and other Asian countries for various conditions, including arthritis, gastrointestinal disorders, liver damage, lymphatic diseases, and various cancers. Recent work has focused on how meshima supports immunity. The mushroom increases the activity of B cells and T lymphocytes, as well as the cytotoxic activity of natural killer cells. Many of meshima's immunologic actions show specific promise for maintaining healthy breast cells.

Meshima mushrooms have been attracting attention as being particularly protective of breast tissue. Researchers from Indiana University found that an extract of meshima suppresses the growth and invasive behavior of breast cancer cells. One of the reasons for the high mortality of breast cancer is the invasive behavior of cancer cells, which results in metastasis (spreading). In the study, reported in the *British Journal of Cancer*, Daniel Sliva, PhD, and colleagues demonstrated that meshima extract (PL-fraction) inhibits proliferation as well as colony formation of highly invasive breast cancer cells. The study suggests a potential therapeutic effect of meshima extract against invasive breast cancer.

Meshima has been well-studied by Korean researchers and is becoming increasingly popular as an adjuvant cancer treatment along with chemotherapies. One study found that meshima increased effectiveness against tumor growth and metastasis in mice when combined with the anticancer drug Adriamycin.

Research shows that meshima has strong antitumor properties. A hot-water extract of meshima had the strongest antitumor activity in a group of medicinal mushrooms that included enoki, kawaratake (Coriolus), a relative of reishi (*Ganoderma applanatum*), and shiitake. The effect was measured in a mouse model of a connective-tissue tumor.

Clinical evidence of meshima's antitumor effects are described in the scientific literature. For example, a female breast-cancer patient in her thirties had been suffering from pain due to a tumor the size of a table-tennis ball near her rib after removal of her left breast. Two months after she began using meshima, the tumor disappeared.

Another report describes an elderly patient who experienced spontaneous cancer remission, a rare phenomenon. A seventy-nine-year-old Japanese man was admitted to a hospital complaining of abdominal discomfort. An MRI and CT scan revealed a liver tumor that was three centimeters in diameter and multiple lung metastases. The patient's medical history showed that he had been treated previously for recurring chronic hepatitis C and liver cirrhosis. After receiving the cancer diagnosis at the hospital, the patient followed up with another physician, but no therapy was performed. Independently, he decided to take a meshima extract for one month. Six months later, a follow-up MRI and CT scan showed no signs of the liver tumor or the chest lesions. The patient continues to be monitored, and further medical imaging shows no recurrence of the cancer after ten months.

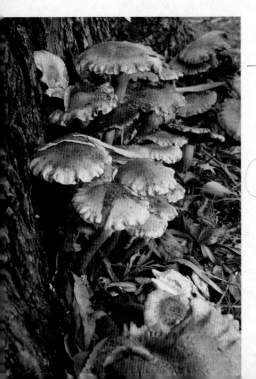

Reishi *Mushroom of Immortality*

Reishi (*Ganoderma lucidum*) is called the "mushroom of immortality" and has been consumed in China for two thousand years as an antiaging herb and to improve the capacity of the mind and memory. In several studies, reishi has been reported to significantly increase the life span of fruit flies by 16 to 17 percent. It is said to be a supreme *shen* (spiritual) tonic that invokes peacefulness, strengthens nerves, and changes how we perceive life. Conditions associated with disturbed *shen* include excessive mental activity, heart palpitations, insomnia, and stress.

Science validates many of reishi's positive health effects, which are extremely broad. Studies support its use for various conditions that can be grouped under several bodily systems, including the cardiovascular system (coronary heart disease, high blood fats, hypertension), immune system (bacterial and viral infections and cancer), and respiratory system (allergies and bronchitis).

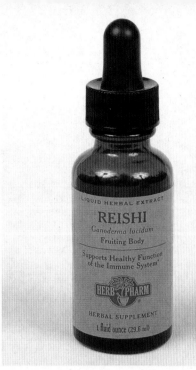

Reishi has approval in Japan for treating certain types of cancers and has been used safely and effectively in conjunction with drugs or radiation. According to Memorial Sloan-Kettering Cancer Center, reishi has been demonstrated to stimulate the immune system in patients with advanced cancers. One study showed that reishi significantly inhibited the growth of leukemia cells.

Reishi has double-direction activity, which means it improves functioning of the immune system whether it is deficient or overactive. It doesn't stimulate the immune system; rather, it regulates it. Therefore, reishi is considered an immune modulator. In Japan and China, it has been approved for treating myasthenia gravis, a serious autoimmune disorder.

Reishi is widely used in Asia to support cardiovascular functions and to reduce LDL cholesterol. It has been found to be effective in preventing and treating angina, arteriosclerosis (hardening of arteries), and shortness of breath associated with coronary heart disease.

In Chinese clinical studies, more than two thousand patients with chronic bronchitis were treated with reishi. Within two weeks, 60 to 90 percent of patients showed significant improvement, with older patients and those with asthma benefiting most. In test tube experiments, compounds contained in reishi have been shown to be effective against influenza A.

Ganoderic acids in reishi inhibit histamine release (allergic reactions), improve oxygen utilization and endurance, support liver functions, and scavenge free radicals. In Tibet, Himalayan guides use reishi to help combat high-altitude sickness. Chinese mountain climbers who took reishi before ascending mountains as high as seventeen thousand feet experienced minimal reactions to the climbs.

A study found that reishi extracts compared favorably with prednisone, a common steroidal anti-inflammatory drug with potentially serious side effects. Reishi had few, if any, negative side effects.

Reishi has an unusual application of being used as an antidote for poisonous mushrooms. It also is an excellent choice as an antistress herb to ease tension. It has been used routinely by monks, sages, shamans, and spiritual seekers. Many people who take reishi regularly notice that it brings peacefulness, an effect that cannot be explained by science.

Shiitake *Most Popular Exotic Mushroom*

Shiitake (*Lentinus edodes*) is Japan's number one agricultural export and the most cultivated, popular, and researched exotic mushroom in the

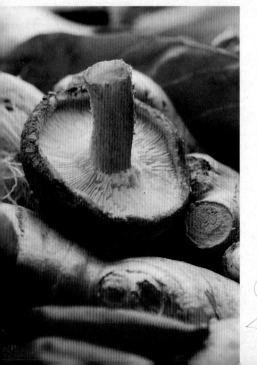

world. *Take* is Japanese for mushroom, and *shii* refers to the kind of chestnut tree on which the mushroom commonly grows. Many gourmet cooks prefer the more delicious, exotic taste of shiitake compared to that of the common and somewhat bland button mushroom.

In China, shiitake has a history that dates back to the Ming Dynasty (1368–1644 AD). The mushroom was used both as a food and medicine. In Chinese folk medicine, shiitake is recommended to activate blood flow, boost *chi* (energy), and fend off a variety of ailments, including bronchial inflammation, cancerous growths and malignancies, colds, flu, heart trouble, and measles. Shiitake is now used clinically to treat AIDS, allergies, cancer, Candida overgrowth, diabetes, exhaustion, high cholesterol, high blood pressure, and viral disorders.

Initial antitumor research involving shiitake was performed in 1969 by scientists at Purdue University and in Tokyo. The researchers found that water extracts of shiitake and several wild mushrooms produced high rates of tumor inhibition in mice (72 to 92 percent). Researchers later identified a polysaccharide in shiitake called lentinan as having powerful immunologic activity.

Shiitake is recognized for its antitumor action and is the most researched mushroom in regard to its immunologic activity.

Shiitake is the source of two extensively studied derivatives with pharmacological action: lentinan, an immune system stimulant and anticancer drug used in Japan, and lentinan enodes mycelium extract, a Japanese food supplement. It should be noted that the greatest medicinal efficacy of shiitake lentinan and extract is achieved through intravenous administration, and that higher oral doses are needed to induce positive effects.

A study at the University of Michigan, Ann Arbor, found that shiitake could produce a highly significant level of protection against influenza A, the kind associated with major epidemics. The mushroom performed slightly better in preventing degradation of lung tissue in mice that were exposed to the virus than the anti-influenza drug Amantadine. Further research revealed that shiitake contains viruslike particles that are similar in structure to an influenza virus and are able to stimulate interferon, a virus-fighting protein.

Research demonstrates that shiitake is a promising treatment for high blood pressure and high cholesterol. Human studies have shown that consumption of large amounts of fresh and dried shiitake resulted in cholesterol decreases ranging from 7 to 14 percent.

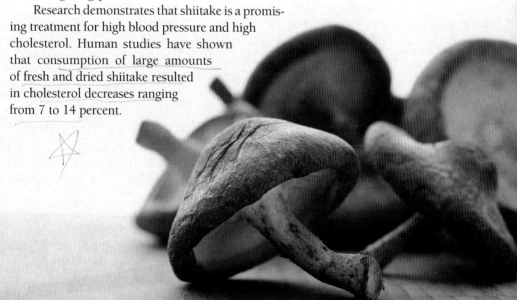

Tremella *Beauty Mushroom*

Tremella fuciformis, also known as white jelly leaf, has a long history of use for nourishing the kidneys, lungs, and stomach and increasing moisture in the body. It is classified as a *yin-jing* tonic, which means it enhances the primal energy of life by helping the body assimilate and store life-giving substances.

Tremella's skin-hydrating properties make it particularly useful as a beauty aid when it is taken either internally and externally. Proper hydration is the main objective of many popular cosmetic ingredients, such as hyaluronic acid (HA), which garnered much attention when it was discovered in the diets of long-lived inhabitants of Yuzurihara, known as "the village of long life," outside of Tokyo. Here, degenerative diseases are rare, and few people show signs of aging in their skin. HA may deter aging by helping cells retain moisture, which keeps the skin smooth and elastic.

Cosmetic companies have recently begun to explore Tremella's promise as a cosmetic aid. When compared to HA, Tremella demonstrated a stronger water-holding capacity (it can hold five hundred times its weight) than sodium hyaluronate, a stable form of HA. Tremella not only moisturized skin better but also helped the skin retain water longer. Tremella mushroom is now a key ingredient in a facial cream called Aquamella. Tremella tablets and skin cream may be used together to maximize this mushroom's ability to nourish skin, inside and out.

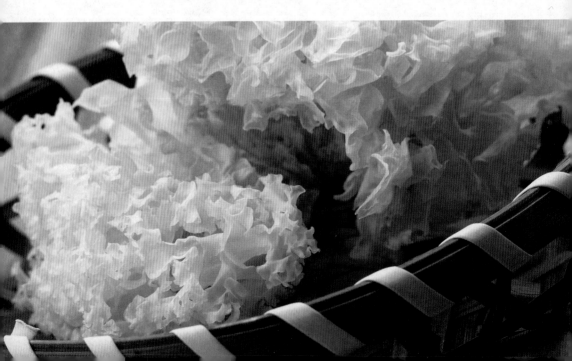

ANCIENT CHINESE SECRET

Some of the best health and beauty discoveries have come out of Asia, where techniques to achieve radiant health and beauty have been practiced for thousands of years. Yang Guifei, the courtesan of an eighth-century Chinese emperor, is said to be the most beautiful woman in Chinese history. Her beauty distracted the emperor from ruling and the country began to fall apart. As the story goes, when she walked through a garden the flowers bowed before her beauty. When asked what her beauty secret was, she replied, "Tremella."

Tremella is popular in Asian cuisine and is one of the oldest cultivated mushrooms. Traditionally, the mushroom was consumed as a delicacy. Because it was rare, it was a luxury available only to the rich.

Tremella is gelatinous and has a nearly white translucent color. The mushroom is composed of 70 percent fiber, which makes it useful for managing cholesterol levels, irregularity, and weight. Tremella contains the highest amount of vitamin D (ergosterol) of all edible natural foods.

In traditional Chinese medicine (TCM), Tremella is used to make a cough syrup for treating asthma, chronic bronchitis, and dry cough. According to TCM, Tremella nourishes the kidneys, lungs, and stomach. In TCM, skin belongs to the lung network, which provides moisture to the skin. Tremella also is believed to remove facial freckles if used frequently.

Tremella is recommended in China for abnormal menstruation, constipation, dysentery, gastritis, and weakness after childbirth. It is said to enhance gonadal activity, reduce fevers, heal ulcers, and promote secretion of saliva. It is administered as a lukewarm preparation made by soaking 3 to 4 grams of the mushroom for one to two hours, cooking it down to a paste, and adding a little sugar to make it taste more appealing. This preparation is taken twice daily.

As is the case for other types of mushrooms, Tremella's immunologic and antitumor activities have gained attention. In one experiment, mice with tumors were fed a diet consisting of 20 percent mushroom powder for one month. The animals were then sacrificed and the weights

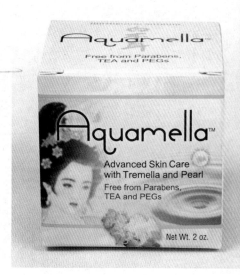

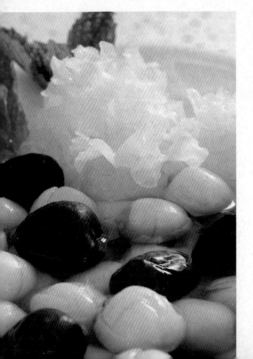

of the growing tumors were measured. Among nine investigated mushrooms, it was found that maitake and Tremella mushrooms had the highest inhibitory activities (86 and 81 percent respectively).

Another study found that when Tremella was administered to mice prior to the transplantation of tumor cells, it had an inhibitory effect on liver and uterine cancers. Survival time was prolonged and survival rate increased. Clinical trials show Tremella is effective in treating leukopenia (loss of white blood cells), which cancer patients experience when undergoing radiation and chemotherapy.

Tremella possesses extensive medicinal potential, including an ability to protect the liver. The mushroom contains polysaccharides that support and protect liver function. Three capsules of Tremella extract (a total of 1 gram) were given daily to forty-five patients with hepatitis for three months. In the thirty-two patients with hepatitis, the success rate was reported to be 56 percent, and in the thirteen patients with chronic persistent hepatitis, it was 77 percent. After treatment, sixteen patients were said to be clinically cured, and after a follow-up period of thirty-six months, fourteen patients were free of further symptoms.

Mushrooms have been investigated as anti-inflammatory agents with low toxicity. Tremella has been proposed as a good candidate. Detailed investigations in lab experiments confirmed Tremella's anti-inflammatory and wound-healing properties when it was administered externally as a paste.

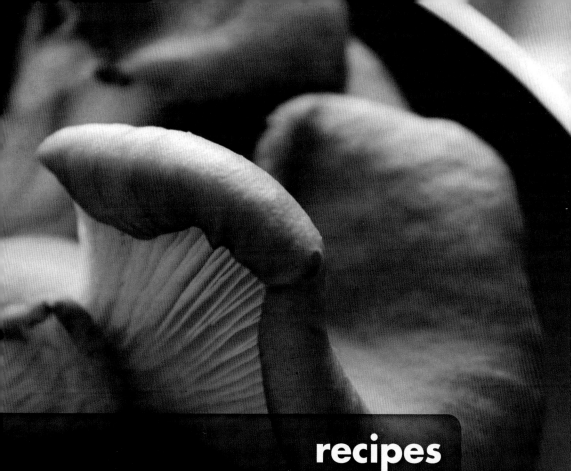

recipes

When shopping, choose firm, fresh-looking mushrooms that are the appropriate size for your recipe. Fresh mushrooms can be loosely wrapped and refrigerated for up to three days. The best way to store them is in a paper bag that has a few holes punched in it. Many types of mushrooms are also available canned or dried.

If fresh mushrooms are to be cooked in liquid, they can be washed. Otherwise, they should be wiped clean with a damp cloth or paper towel. Soaking mushrooms will cause them to absorb too much water and their flavor will be diminished. Peeling mushrooms is unnecessary.

Enoki and Asparagus *soup*

Enoki and asparagus combine well in this elegant soup. Be sure to add the enoki last so that they retain a bit of their crunch. Nutritional yeast flakes provide a boost of nutrition and a chickenlike flavor.

3.5 ounces **fresh enoki mushrooms**

1 pound **asparagus**

6 cups **water or vegetable broth**

1 small **onion, chopped**

5 tablespoons **soy sauce**

1 tablespoon **nutritional yeast flakes**

1 teaspoon **salt**

ground black pepper

3 tablespoons **tapioca starch**

3 to 4 tablespoons **cold water**

Cut off and discard the tough bottoms (about 1 inch) of the mushrooms. Separate the bunches, then separate the mushrooms.

Break off and discard the tough bottom portion of the asparagus and peel the spears. Cut into 1½-inch-long pieces.

Put the water in a large soup pot and bring to a boil over high heat. Add the asparagus, onion, soy sauce, nutritional yeast flakes, salt, and pepper to taste. Decrease the heat to medium, cover, and simmer for 15 minutes.

Dissolve the tapioca starch in the cold water in a measuring cup or small bowl. Stir the dissolved tapioca starch into the soup and cook for 2 minutes, stirring occasionally. Stir in the mushrooms and cook for 2 minutes longer.

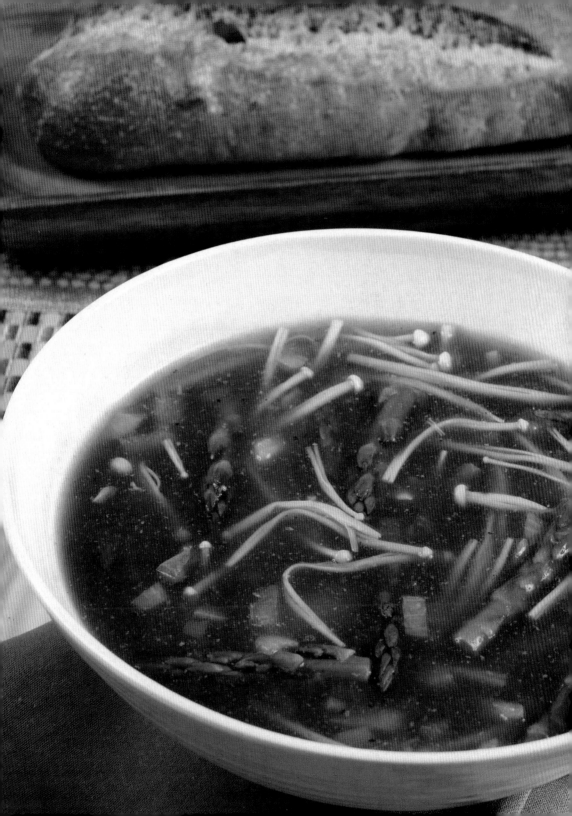

Shiitake and Tofu Clear Noodle *soup*

This light dish will become your favorite new comfort food. Add chili paste if you like it spicy.

8 dried shiitake mushrooms

6 cups water or vegetable broth

1 small onion, finely chopped

1 small carrot, cut into thin matchsticks

3 cloves garlic, finely chopped

3 ounces snow peas, trimmed

4 ounces bean threads

4 ounces extra-firm tofu, cut into 1-inch cubes

chili paste (optional)

salt

ground black pepper

green onion, finely chopped, for garnish

fresh cilantro, for garnish

Soak the mushrooms in warm water for about 10 minutes. Drain. Remove and discard the stems and slice the caps.

Put the water in a large soup pot and bring to a boil over high heat. Add the onion, carrot, and garlic. Decrease the heat to medium, cover, and simmer for 2 minutes. Add the snow peas and mushrooms and cook for 2 minutes. Add the bean threads and cook for 2 minutes, stirring occasionally. Add the tofu and cook for 1 minute longer. Season with chili paste, if desired, and salt and pepper to taste. Garnish with green onion and cilantro.

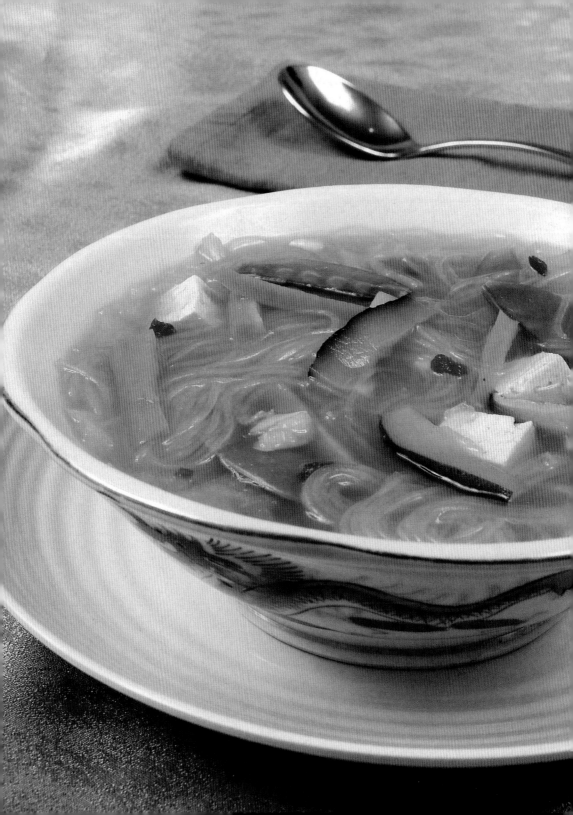

Tremella, Enoki, and Leek *soup*

In Asia, the jellylike Tremella mushroom has been considered a delicacy for thousands of years. In traditional Chinese medicine, Tremella is used as a yin tonic to help hydrate the body's tissues. The Tremella and enoki mushrooms in this soup provide fiber and an exceptional dose of vitamin D.

1.75 ounces **fresh enoki mushrooms**

1 ounce **dried Tremella mushrooms**

4 cups **vegetable broth**

1 small **onion, chopped**

2 cloves **garlic, finely chopped**

4 **leeks, sliced into half-inch rounds**

salt

ground black pepper

Cut off and discard the tough bottoms (about 1 inch) of the enoki mushrooms. Separate the bunches, then separate the mushrooms.

Soak the Tremella mushrooms in warm water for 1 to 2 minutes. Drain. Trim off the tough, discolored bottoms and coarsely chop the tops.

Put the broth in a large soup pot and bring to a boil over high heat. Add the onion, garlic, and Tremella mushrooms. Decrease the heat to medium, cover, and simmer for 2 minutes. Add the enoki mushrooms and leeks. Cover and simmer for 2 minutes longer. Season with salt and pepper to taste.

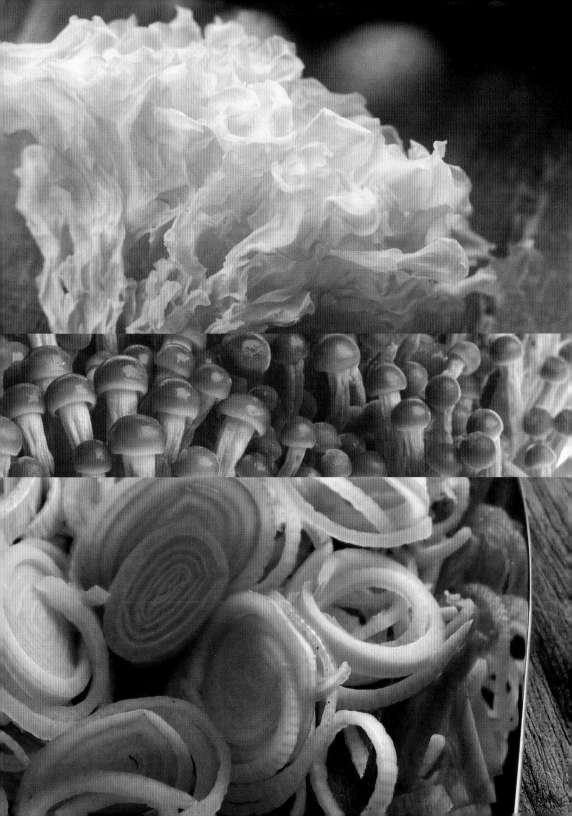

Shiitake, Enoki, and Tofu *spring rolls*

SERVES 4

Enjoy the fresh flavors of mint and cilantro in these spring rolls, which make great finger food for dipping. Serve them for a casual lunch or dinner, or as an appetizer.

SPRING ROLLS

1.75 ounces **enoki mushrooms**

6 fresh large **shiitake mushrooms**, sliced

½ teaspoon **olive oil**

2 ounces **thin rice noodles**

8 large **rice paper wrappers**

6 ounces **prepared fried tofu**, cut into 8 thin slices

4 leaves **romaine lettuce**, cut in half lengthwise, then sliced widthwise into thin strips

chopped **fresh cilantro**

chopped **fresh mint**

To make the spring rolls, cut off and discard the tough bottoms (about 1 inch) of the enoki mushrooms. Separate the bunches, then separate the mushrooms. Cut the mushrooms into thirds.

Fill a small saucepan with water and bring to a boil over high heat. Add the shiitake mushrooms and simmer for 1 minute. Remove the mushrooms with a slotted spoon and set aside. Add the enoki mushrooms to the boiling water and simmer for 1 minute. Drain and set aside.

Fill a medium saucepan with water. Add the oil and bring to a boil over high heat. Add the noodles, decrease the heat to medium-high, and cook for 7 to 10 minutes, or until tender but firm. Drain in a colander. Rinse with cool water and drain again. Let the noodles air-dry.

Pour warm water into a large, shallow bowl until it is half full. Soften each rice paper wrapper, one at a time, just until pliable, by briefly immersing it in the warm water. (Do not allow the wrapper to absorb too much water or it will be difficult to work with.) Transfer the wrapper to a plate. Arrange some of the mushrooms, tofu, noodles, lettuce, cilantro, and mint in a row on the lower third of the wrapper. Carefully fold the bottom edge of the wrapper over the filling. Fold in the sides and continue rolling up from the bottom. Repeat the process with each of the remaining wrappers.

DIPPING SAUCE

3 tablespoons **soy sauce**

2 tablespoons **water**

1 tablespoon **sugar**

2 teaspoons **lemon juice**

½ teaspoon **chili paste**

To make the dipping sauce, combine the soy sauce, water, sugar, lemon juice, and chili paste in a small bowl and mix well. Divide the sauce equally among 4 small serving dishes.

Just before serving, slice each spring roll in half crosswise. Serve with the dipping sauce.

TIP: Prepared fried tofu and rice paper wrappers are available in Asian markets, well-stocked supermarkets, and specialty stores.

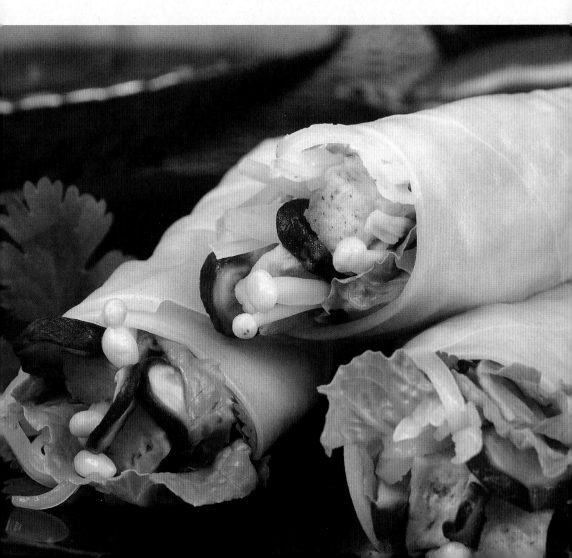

Sautéed Shiitake *mushrooms*

Sautéing shiitake mushrooms is uncomplicated. It only requires a hot pan and some oil to make the most of their smoky, rich flavor. This is one of my favorite ways to prepare them.

8 ounces **fresh shiitake mushrooms**

2 tablespoons **olive oil**

2 cloves **garlic, chopped**

salt

lemon juice

Cut off the mushroom stems and slice them diagonally. Slice the mushroom caps about ¼-inch thick. Heat the oil in a skillet. Add the garlic and cook and stir for about 1 minute, taking care that it doesn't burn. Add the mushroom caps and stems and cook over medium-high heat for about 3 minutes, until they are soft. Add a little more oil if they become too dry. Season with salt and a squeeze of lemon juice to taste.

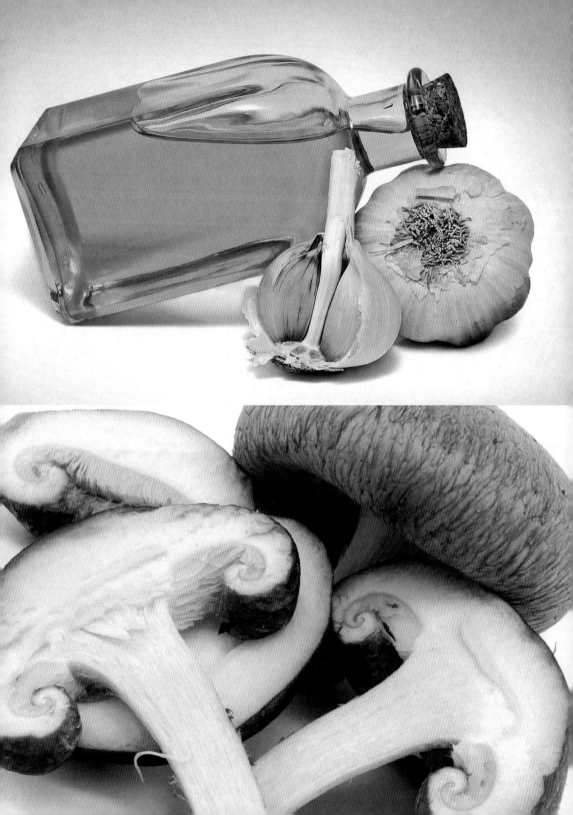

Shiitake-Peanut *tofu*

This is a simple yet flavorful recipe. The shiitake mushrooms, peanuts, and tofu are rich sources of protein. Serve this dish with steamed rice or your favorite whole grain.

1 tablespoon **olive oil**

1 small **onion**, chopped

3 **garlic cloves**, finely chopped

10 fresh small or medium **shiitake mushrooms**, whole

8 ounces **extra firm tofu**, cut into 1-inch cubes

2 tablespoons **soy sauce**

½ cup shelled **roasted peanuts**

salt

ground black pepper

Put the oil in a large skillet or wok over medium-high heat. Add the onion and garlic and cook and stir for 2 to 3 minutes, or until soft. Add the mushrooms and cook and stir over medium heat for 2 minutes. Add the tofu and soy sauce and stir gently. Cover and cook for 2 minutes. Stir in the peanuts, taking care not to break apart the tofu cubes. Cover and cook for 2 minutes longer. (If the mixture is too dry, add a few tablespoons of hot water to moisten.) Season with salt and pepper to taste.

VARIATION: Use ½ cup roasted cashews or almonds instead of the peanuts.

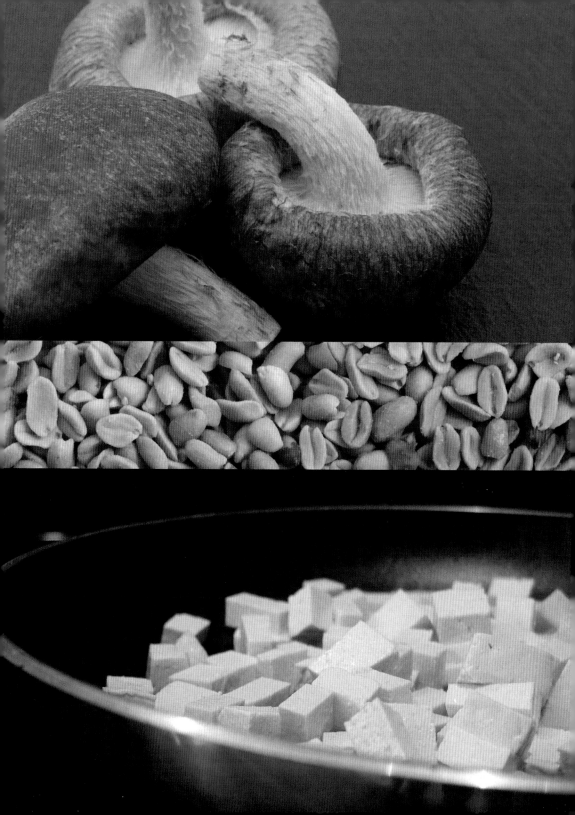

stir-fried vegetables
with Tofu, Maitake, and Enoki

Even people who don't love vegetable will enjoy this hearty Asian-style dish.

1.75 ounces **enoki mushrooms**

2 tablespoons **olive oil**

2 tablespoons finely chopped **onion**

3 cloves **garlic**, finely chopped

2 **carrots**, thinly sliced on a diagonal

2 stalks **celery**, thinly sliced on a diagonal

½ cup peeled and sliced **broccoli stems**

2 tablespoons **hot water**

½ cup **broccoli florets**

½ cup very thinly diagonally sliced **zucchini**

2 ounces **snow peas**, trimmed

6 ounces **prepared fried tofu**, cut into ¼-inch-thick pieces

3.5 ounces **fresh maitake mushrooms**, trimmed and sliced

soy sauce

salt

ground black pepper

Cut off and discard the tough bottoms (about 1 inch) of the enoki mushrooms. Separate the bunches, then separate the mushrooms. Set aside.

Put the oil in a large skillet or wok over medium-high heat. Add the onion and garlic and cook and stir for 2 minutes, or until soft. Add the carrots, celery, and broccoli stems and cook and stir for 1 minute. Add the hot water, cover, and cook for 2 minutes. Stir in the broccoli florets, zucchini, and snow peas. If the vegetables are sticking to the skillet, add a little more hot water. Cover and cook for 2 minutes. Stir in the tofu, enoki mushrooms, and maitake mushrooms. Season with soy sauce, salt, and pepper to taste. Cover and cook for 1 minute longer.

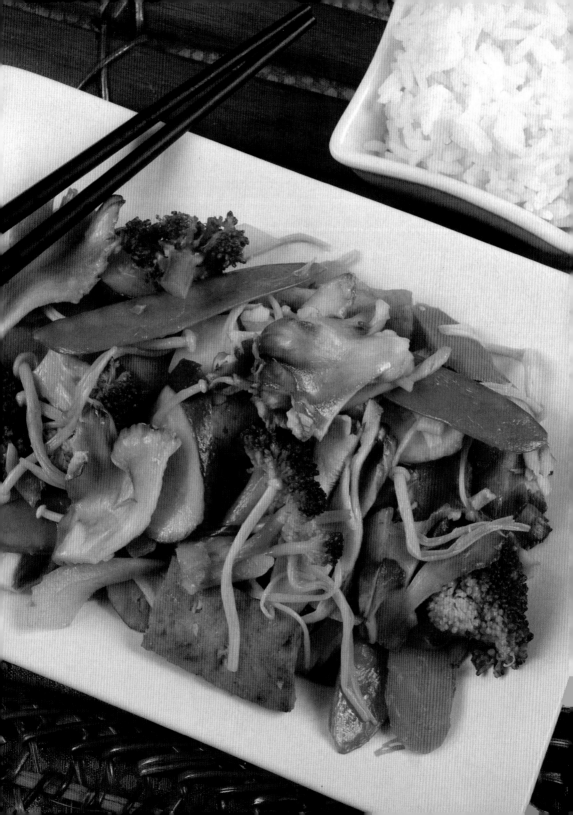

Shiitake and Bok Choy *stir-fry*

Like shiitake mushrooms, bok choy is a common ingredient in Asian cuisine. Its crisp white stems and dark green leaves add a hearty flavor to dishes. Bok choy and other cruciferous vegetables, such as broccoli and cabbage, are known to be potent cancer fighters.

1 pound **baby bok choy** (about 8)

2 tablespoons **olive oil**

3 cloves **garlic, finely chopped**

1 small **onion, chopped**

2 tablespoons **hot water**

10 fresh medium **shiitake mushrooms, whole**

3 tablespoon **soy sauce**

salt

ground black pepper

Separate the bok choy stalks from the leaves. Keeping them separate, slice the stalks and the leaves into 1-inch pieces.

Put the oil in a large skillet or wok over medium-high heat. Add the garlic and cook and stir for 1 minute. Add the onion and cook and stir for 1 minute. Add the bok choy stalks and hot water and cook and stir for 2 minutes. Add the mushrooms and cook and stir for 2 minutes. Add the bok choy leaves and cook and stir for 2 minutes. Stir in the soy sauce. Season with salt and pepper to taste.

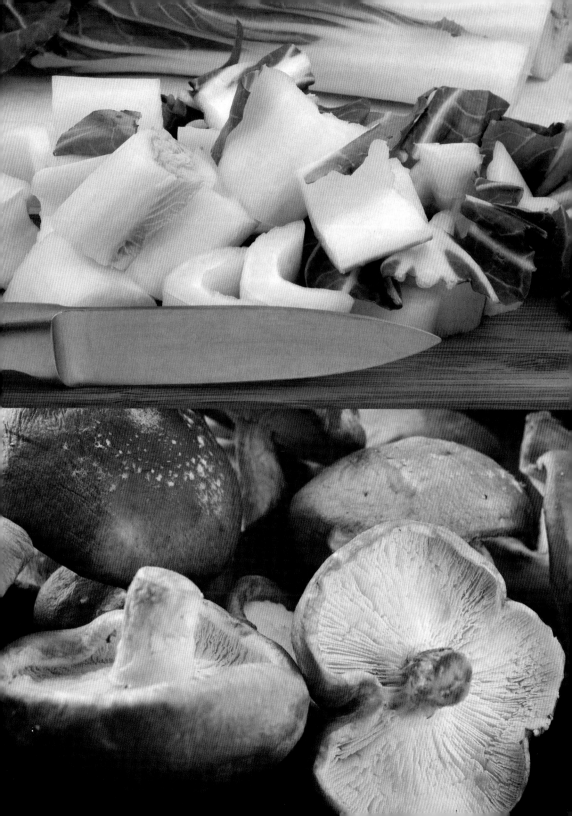

Maitake-Tofu *chow mein*

This is a hearty recipe that satisfies big appetites.

4 tablespoons **olive oil**

2 tablespoons finely chopped **onion**

3 cloves **garlic,** finely chopped

1 large stalk **celery,**
thinly sliced on a diagonal

1 small **carrot,** cut into thin matchsticks

2 ounces **snow peas,** trimmed

1 small **zucchini,** cut into matchsticks

6 ounces **chow mein noodles,**
cooked per package directions and drained

4 ounces **prepared fried tofu,**
cut into ¼-inch-thick slices

3.5 ounces **fresh maitake mushrooms,** trimmed

3 tablespoons **soy sauce**

salt and ground black pepper

Put 3 tablespoons of the oil in a large skillet or wok over medium-high heat. Add the onion and garlic and cook and stir for 1 minute. Add the celery and carrot and cook and stir for 2 minutes. Add the snow peas and cook and stir for 1 minute. Add the zucchini and cook and stir for 1 minute. Add the noodles, tofu, mushrooms, soy sauce, and the remaining tablespoon of oil. Season with salt and pepper to taste. Stir well and cook, stirring occasionally, for about 5 minutes longer.

VARIATION: Use 6 ounces of ramen noodles instead of the chow mein noodles. Cook according to the package directions and drain before using.

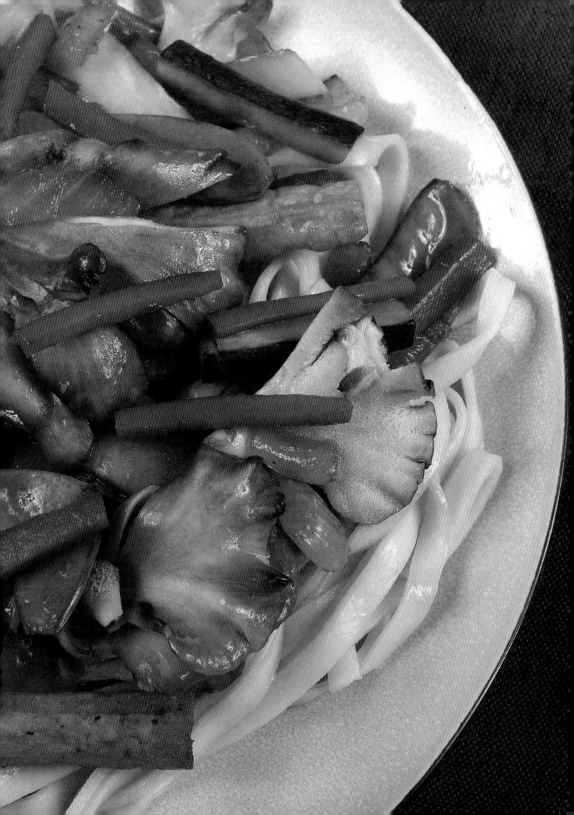

Red Bean and Tremella Mushroom *dessert*

You might not expect to find mushrooms and beans in your dessert. However, in Asian cuisine, Tremella mushrooms and red beans (also called adzuki beans) are common ingredients in all sorts of nutritious desserts.

¾ cup **dried red beans (adzuki beans)**

2 cups **cool water**

½ ounce **dried Tremella mushrooms**

2 cups **hot water**

½ cup **sugar**

1 teaspoon **vanilla extract**

½ teaspoon **salt**

Put the beans in a medium bowl. Cover them with water by 2 inches and let soak for 8 to 12 hours. Drain.

Put the cool water in a medium saucepan and bring to a boil. Add the beans, decrease the heat to medium, cover, and cook for 30 to 40 minutes, or until tender. Add more water as necessary to keep the beans covered. Drain.

Soak the mushrooms in warm water for 1 minute. Drain. Trim off the discolored bottoms and cut the tops into 1-inch pieces.

Add the hot water, mushrooms, and sugar to the beans. Cook for about 15 minutes, stirring occasionally. Stir in the vanilla extract and salt. Remove from the heat and let cool. Cover and refrigerate until thoroughly chilled. Serve cold.

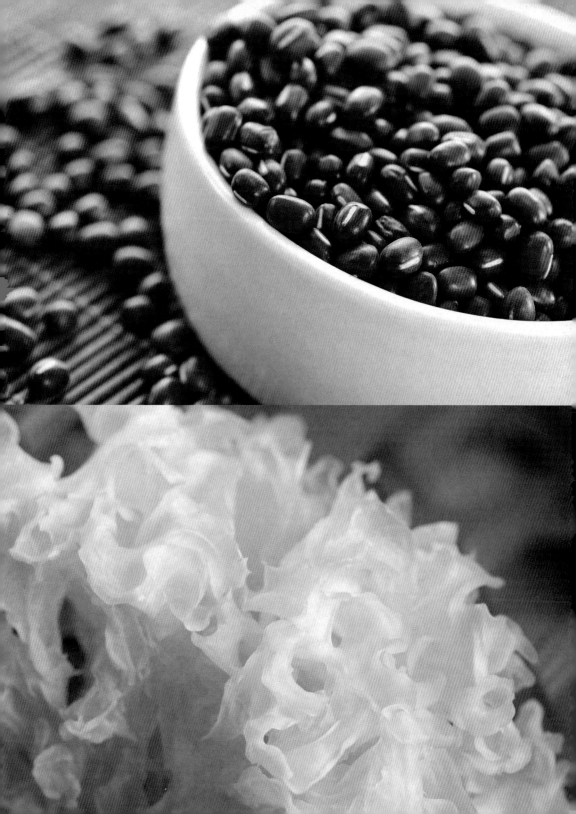

Tremella Tapioca *pudding*

Although mushrooms may seem like an unusual ingredient for a dessert, Tremella mushrooms are slightly sweet and have a jellylike texture that lends itself to dishes like this refreshing pudding.

½ ounce **dried Tremella mushrooms**

4½ cups **water**

4 tablespoons **tapioca pearls**

½ cup **sugar**

1 teaspoon **vanilla extract**

Fresh mint, for garnish

Soak the mushrooms in warm water for 1 minute. Drain. Trim off the discolored bottoms and coarsely chop the tops.

Put 3 cups of the water in a medium saucepan and bring to a boil. Add the mushrooms, decrease the heat to medium, and simmer for 15 to 20 minutes, or until the mushrooms are fairly soft. Add the remaining 1½ cups of water and the tapioca pearls and cook for 15 to 20 minutes, stirring frequently, until the mixture becomes thick. Add the sugar and vanilla extract and cook and stir for 5 minutes longer. Remove from the heat and let cool. Transfer to a storage container, cover, and refrigerate until thoroughly chilled. Serve cold, garnished with fresh mint.

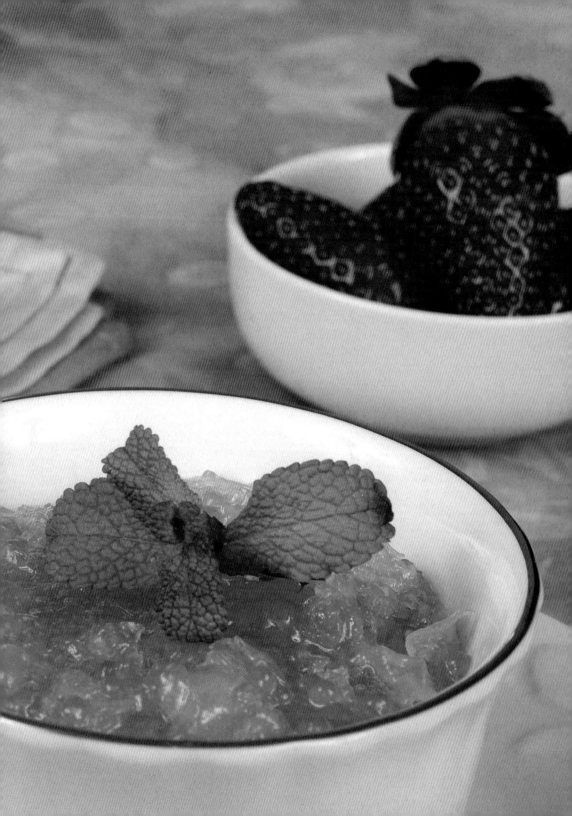

MUSHROOM TERMINOLOGY

Beta glucans. Beta glucans are polysaccharides (linked sugars) that stimulate cellular immunity.

Flush. A flush is the period of time during which large numbers of mushrooms appear all at once.

Fungus. A fungus is a single-celled or multicellular organism that obtains food by direct absorption of nutrients and often produces fruiting (mushroom) bodies.

Gill. Gills are platelike structures on the underside of mushroom caps.

Hyphae. Hyphae are fungal fibers that take in food. As a group, they make up mycelium.

Mushroom. A mushroom is the reproductive fruiting body of a fungus, just as an apple is the reproductive fruiting body of a tree.

Mycelia. Mycelia are the rootlike structures that grow beneath the surface of the growth medium.

Mycology. Mycology is the study of mushrooms and other fungi.

Sclerotia. Sclerotia is a hardened mass of mycelium.

Spore. A spore is a reproductive body that travels through the air; it is similar to a plant's seed.

Toadstool. A toadstool is a poisonous or inedible mushroom.

Yeast. Yeast is the unicellular fungi of the genus Saccharomyces and related genera. It reproduces by budding and is capable of fermenting carbohydrates.

Chen, J. et al. 2010. "Maitake Mushroom (*Grifola frondosa*) Extract Induces Ovulation in Patients with Polycystic Ovary Syndrome: A Possible Monotherapy and a Combination Therapy after Failure with First-Line Clomiphene Citrate." *Journal of Alternative and Complementary Medicine* 16(12): 1–5.

Hayakawa, K. et al. 1993. "Effect of Krestin (PSK) as Adjuvant Treatment on the Prognosis after Radical Radiotherapy in Patients with Non-Small Cell Lung Cancer." *Anticancer Research* 13:1815–1820.

Hong, K. et al. 2004. "Effects of *Ganoderma lucidum* on Apoptotic and Anti-inflammatory Function in HT-29 Human Colonic Carcinoma Cells." *Phytotherapy Research* 18:768–770.

Jones, K. "Maitake. A Potent Medicinal Food." *Alternative and Complementary Therapies*, December 1998, 420–429.

Kawagishi, H. et al. 2009. "Antidementia Effects of a Low Polarity Fraction Extracted from *Hericium erinaceum*." Abstracts of the Fifth International Medicinal Mushroom Conference (pages 18–19), Nantong, China, Sept. 5–8.

Konno, S. 2001. "Maitake SX-Fraction. Possible Hypoglycemic Effect on Diabetes Mellitus." *Alternative and Complementary Therapies*, December, 366–370.

Mizuno, T., C. Zhuang, et al. 1999. "Antitumor and Hypoglycemic Activities of Polysaccharides from Sclerotia and Mycelia of *Inonotus obliquus*." *International Journal of Medicinal Mushrooms* 1:301–316.

Reshetnikov, S. et al. 2000. "Medicinal Value of the Genus *Tremella* Pers. (Heterobasidiomyces) (Review)." *International Journal of Medicinal Mushrooms* 2:169–193.

Sliva, D. 2008. "*Phellinus linteus* Suppresses Growth, Angiogenesis, and Invasive Behaviour of Breast Cancer Cells through the Inhibition of AKT Signalling." *British Journal of Cancer* 98:1348–1356.

Steinkraus, D. C., and J. Whitfield. 1994. "Chinese Caterpillar Fungus and World Record Runners." *American Entomologist* 40 (Winter): 235–239.

Suzuki, F. et al. 1979. "Antiviral and Interferon-Inducing Activities of a New Peptidomanan, KS-2, Extracted from Culture Mycelia of *Lentinus edodes*." *Journal of Antibiotics* 32:1336–1345.

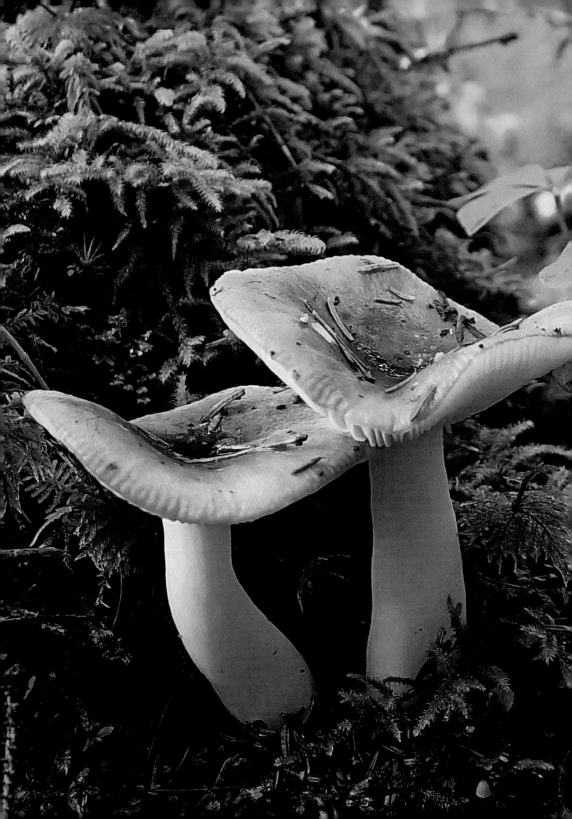

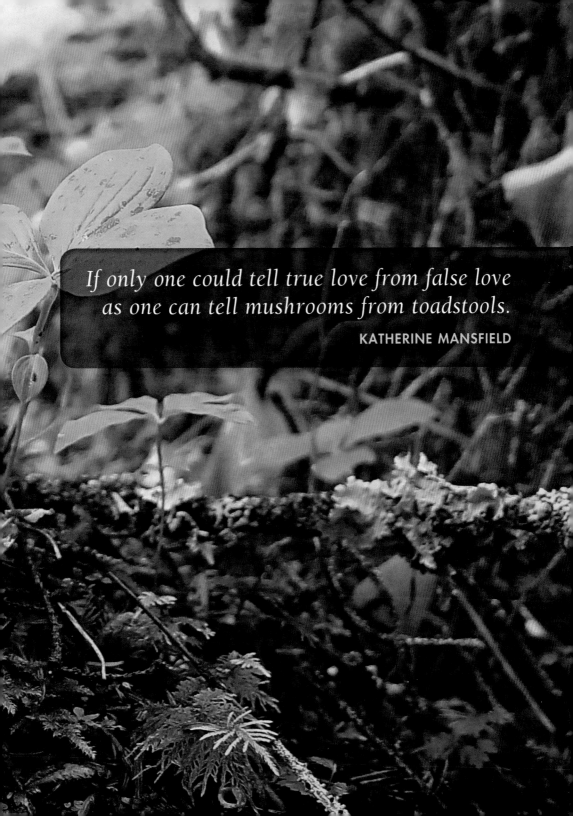

If only one could tell true love from false love as one can tell mushrooms from toadstools.

KATHERINE MANSFIELD

RESOURCES

Herb Pharm
www.Herb-Pharm.com

Jarrow Formulas
www.Jarrow.com

Ken Babal, CN
www.NutritionMusician.com

Mushroom Wisdom
www.MushroomWisdom.com

Phillips Mushroom Farms
www.PhillipsMushroomFarms.com

ABOUT THE AUTHOR

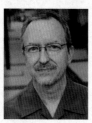

Ken Babal is a consultant to the natural food and supplement industry and has a nutrition counseling practice in Los Angeles. He is the author of several books, including *Seafood Sense: The Truth about Seafood Nutrition and Safety & Maitake Mushroom and D-Fraction.* He is also the author of the Alive Natural Health Guide *Good Digestion: Your Key to Vibrant Health.*

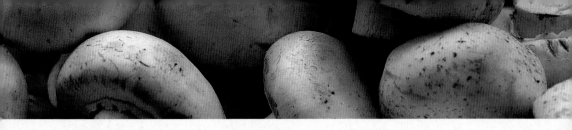

Published by **Books Alive**
PO Box 99
Summertown, TN 38483
931-964-3571
888-260-8458
www.bookpubco.com

Recipes: Cam-Tu Nguyen
Food photography: Warren Jefferson
Food styling: Ron Maxen, Warren Jefferson
Book design, photo editing: John Wincek
Editing: Beth Geisler, Jo Stepaniak

Library of Congress Cataloging-in-Publication Data

Babal, Ken.
    Mushrooms for health and longevity / Ken Babal,.
        p. cm.
    Includes bibliographical references and index.
    ISBN 978-1-55312-047-6
  1. Mushrooms—Therapeutic use.   I. Title.
    RM666.M87B33 2011
    615.9'5296—dc22

                            2011005864

ISBN: 978-155312-047-6

Printed in Hong Kong

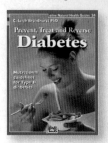 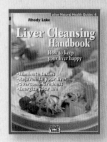 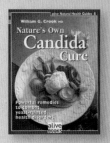
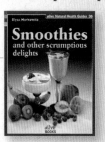 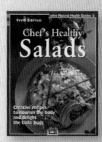 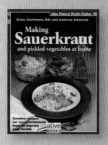
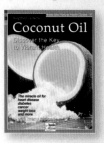 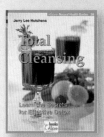 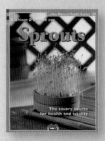
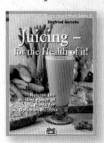 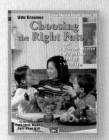 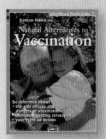